The Diverticulitis Mastery Bible: Your Blueprint For Complete Diverticulitis Management

Dr. Ankita Kashyap and Prof. Krishna N. Sharma

Published by Virtued Press, 2023.

THE DIVERTICULITIS MASTERY BIBLE: YOUR BLUEPRINT FOR COMPLETE DIVERTICULITIS MANAGEMENT

First edition. November 20, 2023.

ISBN: 979-8223760917

Written by Dr. Ankita Kashyap and Prof. Krishna N. Sharma.

Table of Contents

DISCLAIMER

The information provided in this book is intended for general informational purposes only. The content is not meant to substitute professional medical advice, diagnosis, or treatment. Always consult with a qualified healthcare provider before making any changes to your diabetes management plan or healthcare regimen.

While every effort has been made to ensure the accuracy and completeness of the information presented, the author and publisher do not assume any responsibility for errors, omissions, or potential misinterpretations of the content. Individual responses to diabetes management strategies may vary, and what works for one person might not be suitable for another.

The book does not endorse any specific medical treatments, products, or services. Readers are encouraged to seek guidance from their healthcare providers to determine the most appropriate approaches for their unique medical conditions and needs.

Any external links or resources provided in the book are for convenience and informational purposes only. The author and publisher do not have control over the content or availability of these external sources and do not endorse or guarantee the accuracy of such information.

Readers are advised to exercise caution and use their judgment when applying the information provided in this book to their own situations. The author and publisher disclaim any liability for any direct, indirect, consequential, or other damages arising from the use of this book and its content.

By reading and using this book, readers acknowledge and accept the limitations and inherent risks associated with implementing the strategies, recommendations, and information contained herein. It is always recommended to consult a qualified healthcare professional for personalized medical advice and care.

Introduction

The Diverticulitis Mastery Bible: Your Blueprint for Complete Diverticulitis Management

Introduction

By Dr. Ankita Kashyap

1. State the Problem:

Millions of people worldwide suffer from diverticulitis, which significantly lowers their quality of life and causes pain and discomfort. Diverticula are tiny pouches that grow in the colon's lining and become inflamed or infected when the disorder affects the digestive system. Diverticulitis can strike anyone, although people over 40 are more likely to get it.

2. Paint the Picture:

Diverticulitis has a significant effect on people. It ruins everyday schedules, restricts physical activity, and frequently results in episodes of excruciating pain and misery. Diverticulitis can cause mild to severe symptoms, such as fever, bloating, altered bowel motions, stomach pain, and even complications including perforations or abscesses. These symptoms have an adverse effect on mental health as well as physical health, contributing to stress, anxiety, and depression.

Moreover, diverticulitis has a profound effect on society at large. As more people seek medical attention and, in more serious cases, end up in hospitals, the expense of healthcare goes up. It also has an impact on productivity at work, which leads to missing work and poorer output. Diverticulitis has an impact on families, communities, and healthcare systems in addition to the individual.

3. Personalize the Problem:

Sarah is a 45-year-old woman who has been battling diverticulitis for a number of years. Allow me to introduce her to you. Sarah used to be a dynamic, busy person who lived life to the fullest and was constantly on the go. But after receiving her diagnosis, she has had to drastically alter her way of living. Her inability to participate in physical activities due to the regular episodes of abdominal pain and discomfort has made her feel alone and cut off from the outside world.

Sarah's mental health has been impacted by her disease as well. She frequently experiences anxiety and depression because she worries about the effects of the next flare-up on her day-to-day activities. She has a network of friends and relatives who are supportive, but she still feels alone in her problems and misunderstood at times. Her general contentment and sense of fulfilment have suffered as a result of her ongoing anxiety and physical restrictions.

4. Highlight the Stakes:

Diverticulitis can cause serious side effects including abscesses, perforations, or fistulas if it is inadequately handled or left untreated. These issues can potentially be fatal, so you should get medical help right now. Furthermore, one cannot ignore the effect on mental health. Constant discomfort, agony, and limits can lower one's quality of life and exacerbate depressive, anxious, and isolated sentiments.

Globally speaking, diverticulitis is becoming more and more common, which presents a big problem to healthcare systems. Medical resources are under pressure due to the growing number of patients, possible consequences, and related healthcare expenses. If this issue is not adequately addressed, it may overload the healthcare system, delaying treatment and providing insufficient assistance to those with diverticulitis.

5. Transition to Solution:

Fortunately, those who are suffering from diverticulitis have hope. With a thorough guidebook, The Diverticulitis Mastery Bible: Your Blueprint for Complete Diverticulitis Management, people may take charge of their disease and enhance their general well-being. Insights from my team of specialists in a variety of health and wellness sectors are combined with my experience as a medical doctor and health and wellness coach in this book.

You will find evidence-based knowledge, doable tactics, and helpful hints to effectively manage diverticulitis inside the pages of this book. This book offers a comprehensive approach to managing diverticulitis, including everything from dietary and lifestyle changes to counselling and psychological techniques, self-care alternatives, complementary techniques, self-help strategies, and coping processes.

I think that people can get well overall, feel less depressed, and recover control over their life by treating the underlying causes of diverticulitis and using a holistic approach. My goal is to support you during this journey and arm you with the information and resources you need to prosper in spite of diverticulitis's difficulties.

Let's go out on this life-changing path to total diverticulitis control together. Using the Diverticulitis Mastery Bible as your roadmap, you will learn a comprehensive approach to health and wellbeing that goes beyond treating symptoms and enables you to lead a full life without being constrained by diverticulitis.

Are you prepared to regain control over your life and manage your diverticulitis? Together, let's set off on this voyage.

Understanding Diverticulitis

The Basics of Diverticulitis

As a physician and health and wellness coach, allow me to inform you about a disorder called diverticulitis that has a large name but a significant impact. My responsibility is to inform my patients on the fundamentals of this illness. So grab a seat, for this subchapter will take you deep into the anatomy and physiology of the digestive system. You will have a thorough understanding of diverticulitis and how it affects your body by the end of this, I guarantee you.

Now picture your digestive system as a super team: a sophisticated arrangement of tissues and organs that cooperate to process food, absorb nutrients, and say goodbye to waste. The mouth, oesophagus, stomach, small intestine, large intestine (sometimes called the colon), rectum, and anus are members of this squad. Every hero plays a part in ensuring that your body receives the nourishment it requires to run like a well-oiled machine.

Our journey through the digestive system starts in the mouth, where our storey begins. Picture yourself breaking down your favourite dish into smaller, more manageable pieces with your teeth and combining it with saliva. After that, the partially broken down food passes via the oesophagus, a muscular tube that joins the stomach and the mouth. It resembles an exhilarating rollercoaster!

The stomach will come next! It can be compared to a tiny chemistry lab. Food particles are broken down into chyme, a semi-liquid material, by the stomach fluids, which are equipped with hydrochloric acid and enzymes. Mother Nature is an amazing spicer; you have to give her credit!

But hold on tight—the experience is far from over. The small intestine is where the chyme travels down the digestive tract and becomes the true team MVP. This is the point of magic. The duodenum, jejunum, and ileum are the three portions that make up the small intestine. The nutrients in the chyme are disassembled into their most basic components and absorbed into the bloodstream because of the digestive enzymes and the amazing lining of the small intestine. It's similar to a celebration when your health is enhanced and your cells are nourished!

This brings us to our next topic: the colon, or large intestine. This hero has a task of its own. It is in charge of producing and removing stool as well as reabsorbing water and electrolytes. Imagine a five-foot-long tubular organ that is separated into four portions. The colon essentially fills in like a plumber, ensuring that everything works as it should.

But our narrative doesn't end there. These cunning small pouches called diverticula can occasionally make an unexpected appearance inside the big intestine. They resemble uninvited guests at home. Small, protruding sacs known as diverticula protrude through the colon's weak points in the wall. Although they can form anywhere in the colon, the lower region known as the sigmoid colon appears to be their preference. It's comparable to a hide-and-seek game!

Hold on now. It's not always a bad thing to have these diversionary items nearby. Some fortunate people may even be able to obtain them unknowingly. But let me tell you, my buddy, it's game over when these pouches become inflamed or infected (play the scary music). Diverticulitis then interrupts the celebration.

When the diverticula become inflamed, diverticulitis occurs. It has a variety of symptoms, none of which are enjoyable, believe me. Consider nausea, vomiting, fever, bloating, tenderness and pain in the abdomen, as well as disruptions to your regular bathroom schedule. Suddenly, the ordinary life turns into an unexpected roller coaster.

The gimmick? Diverticulitis can cause more than just bad days. It can lead to some really dangerous things if it is not handled seriously or is badly managed. We are discussing the formation of abscesses, fistulas, obstruction of the gut, and even perforation. It resembles a thriller film in which the stakes are always rising.

Knowing the ins and outs of the digestive tract makes it easier to understand the devastation diverticulitis causes. Through an understanding of the formation process and preferred locations of such diverticula, we can access the underlying mechanisms that lead to diverticulitis. And that understanding? It holds the key to determining the most effective methods for symptom relief, averting problems, and maintaining general health.

We will now delve even more in the upcoming chapter. We'll discuss the various risk factors for diverticulitis, ranging from food habits and lifestyle decisions to genetic susceptibility. With this information at your disposal, you'll be able to make wise decisions regarding your health and wellbeing. Together, let's take on this adventure to become experts at diverticulitis management in order to live longer, better lives.

Symptoms and Warning Signs

So, you can imagine the type of patients I see on a daily basis in my capacity as a medical doctor and health and wellness consultant. Yes, you read correctly: diverticulitis sufferers. And believe me when I say that early detection of those bothersome symptoms can truly make all the difference in the world in terms of effectively managing this ailment.

Diverticulitis, my buddy, is not a fun condition. It's a horrible intestinal condition that causes problems with digestion. As you can see, your colon's muscular wall begins to develop small pouches known as diverticula all over the place. And these pouches form when the pressure weakens those areas. Seems harmless enough, doesn't it? But here's the real deal: you're going to experience excruciating agony and discomfort if these pouches get infected or inflamed.

Abdominal pain is one of the most typical signs of diverticulitis. And trust me when I say that this isn't your average pain. No, dear! Though it will also try the right side, this little devil prefers to make its home on the lower left side of your abdomen. This discomfort, too? It is similar to a severe, unrelenting cramping feeling. What's the best part, you ask? If you eat, it can even get worse. What a double-edged sword! I promise you, as soon as this pain becomes unbearable and knocks you down, you should call the doctor.

But there's still more! Additionally, diverticulitis tends to interfere with bowel motions. Yes, it can cause constipation, diarrhoea, or even a lovely combination of the two. It can also cause other interesting surprises. Isn't that delightful? You never know what to expect on your excursions to the bathroom; it's like a game of chance. And to make matters worse, occasionally you may even notice some blood in your stools. Indeed, not precisely what you wanted to see.

Let's now discuss fevers. Your body enters full combat mode when your small diverticular friends get infected. How does it demonstrate that it means business? By raising your body temperature, my companion. These fevers range in temperature from a summer barbecue to a leisurely Sunday afternoon. Oh, and don't be shocked if you have chills and sweats as well. Isn't it true that diverticulitis like keeping things interesting?

But there's still more! Along for the ride with diverticulitis might be some delightful nausea and vomiting. Your digestive system is interfered with by the inflammation in your intestines, causing your stomach to feel like a rollercoaster. And believe me when I say that you should rush to the doctor as soon as possible if you are having trouble swallowing food or if your vomiting won't stop.

This is where it can get really spooky. Diverticulitis can sometimes result in even more terrifying side effects. Consider an incision or possibly a sepsis formation. Yes, you are correct. Big, fancy terminology for very significant concerns. Your abdominal pain starts to intensify to a completely new degree. Like a race vehicle on steroids, your heart rate increases. If that's not enough, you may even begin to exhibit infection-related symptoms, such as an elevated white blood cell count. True enough, that's when things really become messy.

But, my friend, here's the thing. It's imperative—I mean imperative—to recognise these warning indicators. Don't disregard them. No, don't even consider that. You had better get to your doctor as soon as possible if you experience any of these symptoms—better than waiting for a cheetah to become high on caffeine. The trick is to intervene early. It can enhance your overall result and assist avoid those unpleasant problems. However, keep in mind that not everyone has the same combination of symptoms. You know, diverticulitis likes to throw things a little off.

Let's move on to the topic of prevention, as that requires a different discussion. Diverticulitis can be caused by a few different conditions, while the specific aetiology of the illness is yet unknown. Listen up, then! Consuming a diet deficient in fibre, being overweight, smoking excessively, staying sedentary, and using certain medications, such as expensive nonsteroidal anti-inflammatory drugs, can all increase your risk of developing diverticulitis. And let's face it, nobody desires to be a member of that group.

But there is hope, so do not be afraid, my buddy. By managing your health, you can lower your chance of contracting diverticulitis. It all comes down to a few simple lifestyle adjustments. Start by adding some high-fiber foods to your diet to bulk it out. Your bowels will appreciate it, I promise. Get up from the couch and move around. Your new best friend is exercise. Hey, why not lose a few pounds and stop smoking those disgusting cigarettes while you're at it? Yes, it's easier said than done, but your stomach will always be appreciative.

Here's the summary, then. It is imperative to identify the warning signs and symptoms of diverticulitis. Don't ignore them. Any of these symptoms—abdominal discomfort, bowel movements, fevers, nausea, and vomiting—should raise the alert and seek medical attention. But don't worry, buddy. By being aware of the triggers and implementing the required lifestyle adjustments, you can take charge of your health and prevent diverticulitis.

And pay attention, for in the upcoming chapters I will impart some very important knowledge. We're going to get into all the juicy details, including coping mechanisms, nutrition planning, counselling, psychology, and lifestyle adjustments. By working together, we can conquer diverticulitis and regain control of our health. Feel good? I anticipated your support. Let us proceed!

Risk Factors and Triggers

Alright, visualise this: you are ageing, correct? It is undeniable. Additionally, ageing brings with it some less enjoyable things, such as weakened colon walls. Yes, you did hear me correctly. The colon walls seem to be saying, "Hey, let's make some fun stuff!" At that point, diverticulitis actually poses a threat. But wait—being older does not guarantee that you will develop this illness. There are additional variables involved, such as your general health and lifestyle decisions.

Let's now discuss your diet. Watch out if it's poor in fibre! Diverticula can form when a diet high in refined carbohydrates and processed foods, such as those gourmet potato chips, is consumed. For a digestive system to be happy and healthy, fibre is essential. It gives your stool more weight, which keeps everything going smoothly, if you get what I mean. However, a lack of fibre makes your faeces hard and resistant, which puts strain on your colon. And you know what? Diverticulitis, also known as diverticula, can result from that pressure.

And drink lots of water, my friend. It's significant. That water needs to be kept flowing. It maintains regular digestion and softens stools. Constipation results from your stool becoming dry and irritable due to dehydration. Do you understand what that implies? Increased intestinal pressure can lead to an increase in diverticula and possibly even episodes of diverticulitis.

But there's still more! Let's discuss inactivity and obesity. These two are known to cause problems when it comes to diverticulitis. Your colon is not thrilled when you're dragging around additional weight or when you're just sitting around binge-watching Netflix. Its internal pressure rises, which facilitates the formation of diverticula. Thus, get up from the couch and move! Exercise on a regular basis helps you maintain proper digestion and weight control. Your colon will appreciate it, I assure you.

Okay, let's talk about some unhealthy behaviours now. Smoking while having a good time? They are detrimental to your general health and increase your chance of diverticulitis. Excessive alcohol use aggravates your digestive tract, and smoking has been connected to those bothersome diverticula. So, my friend, it's time to break those bad behaviours. There will be a sigh of relief for your colon.

And listen up if you're struggling with long-term health issues like obesity, diabetes, or hypertension. You have a higher chance of developing diverticulitis. Your body's ability to fight off inflammation and infections is hampered by these diseases, which also interfere with your immune system. To reduce your risk of diverticulitis, it's critical to manage these illnesses and adopt good lifestyle choices. You can do this!

The worst part is that several drugs and treatments might also increase your risk of diverticulitis. Yes, even drugs that seem harmless to take, like aspirin and ibuprofen, can cause inflammation by interfering with the lining of your colon. Additionally, be cautious while undergoing procedures like barium enema or colonoscopy, as these may harm your colon and increase your risk of developing diverticulitis. Before undergoing any of them, make sure you discuss the benefits and drawbacks with your healthcare professional.

Let's now discuss triggers. You see, each person has a unique set of factors that might cause an exacerbation of diverticulitis. Your digestive system is involved, much like in a game of hide and seek. Among the frequent offenders are particular foods, stress, and gastrointestinal tract illnesses. Nuts, nuts, popcorn, and high-fat foods are like a ticking time bomb for diverticulitis sufferers' inflammation. And let's not even talk about stress. Diverticulitis is just one of the many health problems for which it is known to be problematic. Stress exacerbates inflammation and interferes with digestion. Not to be overlooked are those unpleasant gastrointestinal infections. Viral or bacterial invasions have the potential to exacerbate the inflammation in your unlucky colon and result in an episode of diverticulitis.

You must thus be a detective. Determine the cause of your diverticulitis. Record your symptoms in a journal, taking note of any patterns or possible triggers. This will enable you to masterfully prevent those flare-ups and keep one step ahead. Collaborate carefully with your medical professional as well. They will assist you in creating a customised management strategy that will greatly simplify your experience with diverticulitis.

In short, you have to know your opponent, which in this case happens to be the diverticulitis risk factors and triggers. Age is an influence, certainly, but not the only one. You run the risk of developing diverticulitis due to a number of factors, including your food, water intake, exercise routine, smoking, alcohol use, chronic illnesses, prescription drugs, and medical procedures. Furthermore, GI illnesses, stress, and specific foods might exacerbate diverticulitis that has already been diagnosed. But don't worry! You can significantly lower your risk by changing your lifestyle to include eating more fibre, drinking plenty of water, exercising, giving up smoking, and consuming alcohol in moderation. Additionally, by monitoring those triggers and practising stress management and good cleanliness, you can avoid having flare-ups mar your day. Work along with your physician, adhere to your customised treatment plan, and manage your diverticulitis. Boom. You can do this!

Coping With Emotional Impact

You know, having a chronic illness like diverticulitis can really throw you for a loop mentally. You may experience anxiety, tension, and total overwhelm due to the ongoing pain, limitations it places on your everyday activities, and the ongoing fear of a flare-up. And let me tell you, in my opinion—as someone who practises holistic self-care—addressing these psychological and emotional side effects is crucial if I hope to manage my diverticulitis.

First things first, you have to accept and realise that you will experience a wide range of emotions. Experiencing frustration, anger, or just plain overwhelm from all the trash that comes with this disease is quite normal. Allow yourself to feel those emotions rather than suppressing them. Permit yourself to digest and let go of all that bottled-up emotion. Consider keeping a notebook or talking it up with a trusted friend or relative. Hell, you could even try using music or art to express yourself. Simply find a way to express everything.

Be gentle to yourself as well while you're doing it. You must drastically alter your way of living if you have diverticulitis. You may need to modify your diet and abstain from certain activities that may set off another flare-up. To be honest, it can give you the impression that you are losing out on a lot. But hear me out: choosing those options is a self-loving act. "I'm going to take care of myself no matter what," is what you're saying. Thus, try not to be too hard on oneself. Make your health and wellbeing your top priority, and never forget that you have the ability to live your best life even if you have this disease.

Let's now discuss stress. It goes without saying that stress can exacerbate your symptoms and cause a full-blown flare-up. Therefore, learning how to control and lessen stress is crucial. Consider adding some stress-relieving activities to your day, such as yoga, meditation, deep breathing, or engaging in relaxing hobbies. If you make it a habit, you'll experience a significant improvement in your general mood.

Additionally, remember to confide in those who genuinely understand your situation. Look for internet forums or support groups designed just for diverticulitis sufferers. It's incredible how much the knowledge that you're not the only one going through this can lift your spirits. You'll discover acceptance, support, and a safe space to openly discuss your life experiences without fear of repercussions. You can feel so much more at ease and strong with that kind of support, I promise.

Make sure you communicate with your healthcare staff as much as possible. Discuss your emotional struggles with your medical experts, including your doctors. They can provide direction, help you find resources, and provide you with helpful strategies. They may even be able to recommend counsellors or therapists who focus on treating chronic illnesses. The more you discuss it, the more prepared you'll be to deal with the emotional difficulties.

Finally, but just as importantly, you need to strengthen your resilience and maintain a positive outlook. It's easier said than done, I know. It's not easy to have a chronic illness like diverticulitis. Now, though, what? My buddy, you have the ability to thrive despite this because you are adaptive. Begin rephrasing your ideas and convictions, concentrating on life's positive aspects, and cultivating an attitude that genuinely believes you can conquer any challenge. Try keeping a gratitude notebook, picture yourself kicking butt, and say affirmations aloud. Although it may seem corny, it really does wonders.

Hence, addressing the psychological and emotional repercussions of diverticulitis is an important aspect of managing the entire situation. You'll be handling those difficult emotional hurdles like a pro if you can communicate to your healthcare team, be kind to yourself, learn coping mechanisms for stress, lean on others, and embrace and acknowledge your emotions. And never forget that having diverticulitis does not define you. You possess the techniques and mentality necessary to overcome it and have an amazing life.

Support Systems and Resources

I have to be honest with you, listen. Diverticulitis is a serious condition to treat. It's an exhilarating experience that plays havoc with your body and mind. However, believe me when I say that having a strong support network is invaluable.

For those seeking support, establishing connections with like-minded others is an essential component. We are referring to online and in-person support groups. These communities serve as a lifeline, offering a safe space for you to talk about your struggles, ask for help, and connect with others who genuinely get what you're going through. I promise you that it feels like a weight is lifted off your shoulders when you find someone who understands how you truly feel. Additionally, these groups offer you helpful advice on how to manage your symptoms and handle all the complex issues that come with this condition.

During my time as a physician, I have personally witnessed how these support groups provide a secure environment where patients can express themselves without worrying about being judged. It resembles a small village where everyone looks out for one another. It's possible to gain solace, support, and direction from individuals who understand. Just make sure the information is accurate and supported by data. A trusted moderator or a healthcare practitioner in the group can assist steer things in the correct direction.

And remember, there are tonnes of fantastic internet resources available. You must be aware of where to look for trustworthy information. I refer to the websites of organisations such as the American Dietetic Association, the National Institute of Diabetes and Digestive and Kidney Diseases (NIDDK), and the American Gastroenterological Association (AGA) (ADA). These websites are reliable, supported by industry professionals, and offer all the information you require regarding symptom management, available treatments, dietary advice, and lifestyle modifications.

I realise that the internet may be a strange place with a lot of false information. Thus, it's crucial to only use reliable sources. Refrain from clicking on the first link that appears in your Google search. Choose the reliable websites I suggested previously, and you'll be OK. They have all the evidence-based information you require to make wise choices regarding your well-being.

Naturally, we must not overlook the authorities in the domain. It is imperative that you get advice from a gastroenterologist or other specialist in digestive health. These experts can provide you with tailored advice on how to manage your diverticulitis. They will determine the extent of your illness, suggest the best course of action, and provide you with ongoing assistance. Additionally, it's normal for them to recommend alternative practitioners, psychiatrists, or dieticians among other medical specialists. They are all members of the ideal group that will look after you.

Now, though, what? Friends and family can also be superheroes. They are essential in offering both practical and emotional support. They are there to listen, to cheer you up when you're feeling low, and to assist with all the small chores that pile up into major difficulties when flare-ups occur. Just be sure to be honest with them about what you need and what you can't do. They wish to assist, but they are not mind readers. So allow them.

I understand that you may not give self-care and alternate methods much thought, but bear with me. These techniques can significantly improve your general health and aid in symptom management. We are discussing relaxation methods, mindfulness, light exercise, and stress reduction. They can all have a profound impact on how you manage the psychological and physical effects of this illness. But always remember to consult your medical team before beginning. They will ensure that these methods fit into your overall treatment strategy.

Not to mention, never undervalue the effectiveness of coping mechanisms. Keeping a journal, creating art, or taking up a new activity are all excellent ways to treat diverticulitis. They can enhance your wellbeing and serve as emotional outlets.

The bottom line, my friend, is to ask for help, locate trustworthy information, and create a solid support system around yourself. You have supportive friends and family, internet resources, medical professionals that specialise in digestive health, and support groups to help you along the way. Recall that you are not by yourself. Together, we are prepared to overcome diverticulitis. So let us proceed.

Holistic Understanding

You know what's very inconvenient? Diverticulitis. Yes, it's the illness where your colon's tiny pockets known as diverticula get infected and inflamed. It's not a good moment, I can assure you of that.

Now, everyone has heard of the outward signs of diverticulitis, such as bloating, crooked stools, and abdominal pain. However, the role that our emotions and thoughts play in the whole event is something that is frequently ignored.

You see, we have to take the body, mind, and spirit into account when it comes to total well-being. Hey, it's all connected. similar to an enormous network of health. Furthermore, we need to address all aspects of diverticulitis management, including psychological, emotional, and physical issues.

The physical component is quite simple. It's necessary to follow medical advice to manage those symptoms. A change in diet, painkillers, and antibiotics are all essential in treating this illness. The exciting part is that our emotional and mental states can significantly influence how our bodies respond to this beast.

Studies have indicated that stress is a common trigger for a variety of digestive disorders, including diverticulitis. Our bodies go into overdrive when stress strikes, which disrupts our digestive systems. Increased inflammation, digestive problems, and a compromised immune system are all ideal conditions for a resentful colon.

Thus, we also need to address the psychological and emotional issues. Finding a stress-reduction strategy that works for you is key. Deep breathing, meditation, and even taking a relaxing medication might be quite beneficial. Internal serenity can help our bodily symptoms subside and restore our sense of well-being.

However, we must not lose sight of the fact that having diverticulitis can be a true emotional rollercoaster. The psychological effects of chronic pain, anxiety of flare-ups, and overall helplessness can be debilitating. It's crucial to see a therapist or join a support group because of this. They assist you in navigating the emotional rollercoaster, much like guides do. They teach you coping mechanisms, how to dispel negative ideas, and how to maintain an optimistic outlook throughout it all. Living your best life and taking charge are the key components.

Naturally, though, this holistic approach involves more than simply your thoughts and feelings. Baby, this is a whole lifestyle makeover. You must take good care of your physique. Your body may repair and boost its immune system with the support of regular exercise, adequate sleep, and stress-reduction measures. Not to mention the importance of sound diet. To keep your stomach happy and stop flare-ups in the future, you need to eat a diet rich in fibre and nutrients.

While I'm not suggesting that complementary and alternative medicine is the next big thing, they could be useful. Herbal remedies, acupuncture, and all that hippy stuff might be worth a try. Man, it's all about figuring out what suits you.

Therefore, the key to handling this diverticulitis issue is to stand back and consider the wider picture. We are treating the full individual, not just the symptoms. This entails treating the mental, emotional, and physical issues simultaneously. It all comes down to assuming charge and striking a balance that suits you. Well, who knows? Perhaps after this experience, you'll have a completely different outlook on life.

Personal Testimonials

The day seems like it was yesterday to me. The day I learned the phrase diverticulitis, and it completely changed my life. I was forty-five years old, trying to keep up with the demands of life while working nonstop as a professional. Then, whoosh! The diagnosis hit me hard, leaving me reeling from shock and bewilderment.

I can assure you that the pain was unbearable. Those horrible flare-ups seemed like they were tearing apart my insides; they came at me in waves. My standard of living plummeted, and I couldn't help but question if things would ever turn around.

But what's the deal? This is not my first storey. The suffering I experienced is nothing compared to the countless others. Many people are all too familiar with the emotional rollercoaster of anxiety, frustration, and uncertainty that accompanies living with a chronic illness.

But I had to take action. I could not allow this illness to control my life and cause me to continue suffering. I therefore set out on a quest to discover practical methods for controlling my illness. It wasn't easy, I assure you.

People like Dr. Ankita Kashyap gave me comfort and eventually became my guiding light. With her knowledge and the assistance of her multidisciplinary team of professionals, we created a thorough treatment plan just for me. Tailored attention was the deciding factor.

I also changed my way of living, which was really helpful for my recuperation. I bid farewell to trigger foods and adopted a high-fiber diet in order to maintain regular bowel movements and stave off flare-ups. Not to be forgotten is exercise. Adding regular exercise to my routine reduced stress and enhanced my general wellbeing.

And John is the other one. He is another fighter who has long struggled with diverticulitis. His is an inspiring tale of tenacity and willpower. His mental and emotional well being suffered as a result of the unspeakable suffering he experienced. He felt alone and powerless as a result.

However, John resisted letting this illness define who he was. Dr. Kashyap and her colleagues helped him fight back and take back control of his life. He developed coping tools including writing, mindfulness practises, and meditation to help him deal with the stress and anxiety that accompany with diverticulitis.

John's narrative serves as a helpful reminder that we must look after ourselves. Long-term relief from this ailment requires self-care and self-help strategies. And you know what? He even looked into complementary and alternative medicine, which improved his general health.

These aren't just any old stories. They stand for the experiences of many people who suffer with diverticulitis, just like us. We foster a sense of community and provide hope and inspiration to individuals who are feeling overwhelmed by their diagnosis by exchanging personal stories.

See, it's not only about prescription drugs and physicians. An interdisciplinary approach is essential for diverticulitis treatment. The magic happens when medical practitioners from various specialties collaborate to offer holistic care. Customized therapy regimens that are based on the particular requirements and circumstances of each patient are quite beneficial.

Having a chronic illness also has an impact on our psyche and feelings. We learn about the difficulties Sarah and John have faced, the resiliency they have exhibited, and the fortitude it takes to get through it all via their experiences.

These first-hand accounts provide us the confidence to manage our health. We can take the initiative to look for assistance and practical management techniques for diverticulitis. It goes beyond the clinical aspect of things. It's about realising that there is a vibrant community of people who have overcome these obstacles and come out on the other side stronger, smarter, and more prepared to lead happy lives.

In summary, these first-hand accounts provide us with a glimpse into the lives of people who suffer from diverticulitis. They demonstrate for us the difficulties they've encountered, the victories they've acknowledged, and the tactics they've used. They provide encouragement, inspiration, and useful guidance to anyone coping with this illness. They serve as a reminder that we can have happy, healthy lives despite having a chronic condition.

Nutrition and Diet for Diverticulitis Management

Understanding Nutritional Needs

Now, allow me to explain this diverticulitis to you. It resembles the diverticula, which are tiny pouches that appear in the lining of your colon. The best part is that the fun starts when these pouches become infected or inflammatory. You eventually have severe diarrhoea, constipation, bloating, and abdominal pain. Talk about an exciting ride, huh?

Although the actual origin of diverticulitis is yet unknown, a low-fiber diet and an excessive intake of processed foods are suspected to be contributing factors. That whole "you are what you eat" thing, you know? Yes, it is the situation at hand.

Hey, don't worry—there are strategies for controlling this beast. Knowing what your body need in terms of nutrition is crucial. Fiber is also a significant factor in this case. The digestive system's super hero is fibre. It keeps everything in check, keeps everything flowing smoothly, and avoids constipation. Moreover, it has been connected to a decreased incidence of diverticulitis and may help avoid those bothersome flare-ups.

Therefore, maintaining a healthy balance of high-fiber foods in your diet is key. Consider entire grains, legumes, nuts, fruits, and vegetables. Soluble fibre comes in a variety of forms and can be found in foods including beans, apples, and oats. That material absorbs moisture and facilitates the passage of stool. Conversely, insoluble fibre can be found in foods such brown rice, celery, and whole wheat bread. This substance keeps everything flowing and gives your stool more bulk.

But there's still more! Your body also need other vital nutrients. Minerals, vitamins, and antioxidants are all important for maintaining your health and promoting physical healing. Thus, make sure to eat a varied diet that is high in fruits, vegetables, lean proteins, and healthy fats. It's similar like showing your body a little more affection, you know?

This is when things become tough. Certain meals are not compatible with diverticulitis. Certain ones can worsen conditions by causing symptoms. It feels like those cunning little devils are out to get you. Foods heavy in fat, caffeine, alcohol, and spices are the ones that cause problems. In order to identify the foods that are bothering you, keep a look out for those and consider keeping a meal journal. It's similar to playing detective, but instead of cracking cases, you're unravelling the riddle of your stomach.

And inflammation, too. It resembles the antagonist in this tale. Your diverticulitis may worsen due to inflammation, so you should take every precaution to prevent it. The anti-inflammatory diet is now available. Consuming nutritious meals such as almonds, olive oil, berries, leafy greens, and fatty fish is recommended. They aid in reducing inflammation and preventing the symptoms. However, exercise caution as you should avoid artificial additives, saturated fats, and refined sweets. There is no one who wants those men to show up at the party with their inflammation cronies.

As a physician and health and wellness coach, I have now dealt with many patients who have diverticulitis. Furthermore, no two persons are same, I assure you. Every one of us is a different snowflake with distinct dietary requirements, tastes, and tolerances. To create a plan that is ideal for you, it is crucial to collaborate with a nutritionist or healthcare professional. But don't worry, we can work things out together. Together, we will design a customised diet plan, make some lifestyle adjustments, and identify effective coping mechanisms. You, my friend, will be in command.

To put it briefly, the secret to managing diverticulitis effectively is understanding your nutritional requirements. Increase your fibre intake, make sure you're getting all the nutrients you need, avoid trigger foods, and reduce inflammation. By seeking help from experts such as myself, you can take control of your health and make diverticulitis pay for its actions. Let us proceed!

Foods to Embrace

I've been delving deeply into the field of diverticulitis management chapter after chapter. And believe me when I say that a wide variety of foods are available that are quite beneficial for this illness. These foods have incredible qualities that can reduce inflammation, enhance digestion, and hasten healing in addition to being nutrient-dense and full of all the nutrients your body needs. It seems like you have a horde of super heroes waiting to save the day in your kitchen!

My friends, let's start with foods strong in fibre. These little ones are our best friends when it comes to treating diverticulitis. In order to maintain optimal digestive health and avoid uncomfortable constipation that could exacerbate our symptoms, fibre is essential. Consuming fibre gives our faeces more volume (I know, not the prettiest way to say it), which facilitates passage through the intestines and lowers the possibility that anything will become lodged in those bothersome diverticulae.

But there's still more! In actuality, there are two kinds of fibre: soluble and insoluble. In our intestines, soluble fibre absorbs water and forms a gel-like swell that aids in regular bowel movements and guards against diarrhoea. Conversely, insoluble fibre gives our stools more volume and helps us avoid constipation. It is imperative that you incorporate both forms of fibre into your diet as they are genuine heroes when it comes to treating diverticulitis.

Look at these fruits—apples, pears, berries, oranges, and bananas—that are powerhouses of fibre. And believe me, my friends, if you want to really up your fibre intake, you should eat the entire fruit. Additionally high in fibre are vegetables; consider Brussels sprouts, broccoli, cauliflower, carrots, and leafy greens. To get the most out of their fibre goodness, you can roast, stir-fry, add in a salad, or throw them in a soup.

Alright, buddies, let's speak about whole grains. Opt for whole grain superfoods like barley, quinoa, oats, brown rice, and whole wheat bread instead of processed grains. Compared to their refined competitors, these guys are far higher in nutrients and also include a decent quantity of fibre. Good news for all of you who enjoy legumes: chickpeas, peas, lentils, and beans are all amazing sources of high-fiber foods. They can be added to salads, stews, soups, and even used in place of meat. What versatility!

But hold on, my friends—remember to gradually up your fibre consumption. It takes time for your body to adjust, and staying hydrated is essential to preventing any upset stomach. Hold onto that bottle of water!

Let me now introduce the second group of heroes: foods high in probiotics. These men has the ability to cure and reduce intestinal irritation. Probiotics are similar to the good guys in our digestive systems. They aid with digestion, strengthen our immune systems, and maintain the proper balance of bacteria in our intestines. Consuming meals high in probiotics is like arming your stomach with superpowers to fend off inflammation and maintain optimal digestive health.

Yogurt is the first probiotic warrior on our list. Friends, don't settle for any yogurt—search for those with vibrant, living cultures. Here, kefir and Greek yoghurt are excellent options. There are also non-dairy substitutes available, so don't worry if you're on a plant-based diet or are lactose intolerant. Another powerful source of probiotics is sauerkraut. This fermented cabbage-based product is loaded with probiotics. Just be careful to get the unpasteurized variety as the pasteurisation procedure can eliminate those beneficial bacteria. Do you know what kimchi is? It's a classic fermented vegetable dish from Korea. This zesty and hot side dish is rich in vitamins and minerals in addition to probiotics. Not to be overlooked is kombucha, a bubbly, fermented tea beverage that is becoming more and more well-known for its high probiotic content. It can be a welcome and healthy addition to your daily routine and is available in a variety of tastes.

Now, my friends, put on your capes and get ready to meet the next group of heroes: meals high in omega-3 fatty acids. These are vital fats that offer numerous health advantages. However, omega-3 fatty acids are primarily concerned with lowering inflammation and accelerating the healing process in our digestive systems, which is how we treat our diverticulitis.

First up, there are fatty fish, such as trout, sardines, salmon, and mackerel. Make sure to include these fish on your plate at least twice a week as they are a great source of omega-3 fatty acids. My buddies, chia and flaxseeds are small omega-3 powerhouses. To provide a pleasant and nutritional boost to your salads, yoghurt, or cereal, sprinkle them on top. Not to mention, walnuts are a fantastic source of omega-3 fatty acids in addition to being a delicious snack. Add them to your baked products or toss them into salads for a healthy and nutty flavour. Finally, we have tofu and soybeans. These amazing soy-based foods offer a healthy amount of protein along with omega-3 fatty acids. They work well in stir-fries, soups, and even as a meat alternative. Say it with me: delicious.

Let's talk about the third category of superheroes now, my friends: meals that reduce inflammation. When it comes to diverticulitis, inflammation is an unwanted guest, so include these nutrients in your diet to help reduce discomfort and hasten the healing process. These meals are like tiny soldiers, full of substances that combat inflammation in our bodies and antioxidants.

Berries such as blueberries, strawberries, raspberries, and blackberries are powerful anti-inflammatory warriors. These guys are loaded with anti-inflammatory and antioxidant chemicals. Eat them raw, add them to smoothies, or to yoghurt or oatmeal as a topping. My friends, leafy greens like spinach, kale, and Swiss chard are not only high in fibre but also a powerful source of antioxidants. Use them as the base for salads, include them into stews and soups, or sauté them as an accompaniment. Not to be overlooked is turmeric, the vivid yellow spice that contains the incredible substance curcumin. Turmeric is a superfood that helps reduce inflammation, so feel free to incorporate it into soups, curries, and even your homemade golden milk. Finally, but just as importantly, ginger is the calming hero we all need. For generations, ginger has been used to help with digestion and reduce inflammation. It can be steeped into a soothing tea or used to savoury or sweet meals. You're our rock, Ginger!

To sum up, my friends, the food we eat greatly affects the health of our digestive systems. So let's feed ourselves these nutrient-rich warriors and take charge of managing our diverticulitis. Foods high in fibre, rich in probiotics, foods high in omega-3 fatty acids, and foods low in inflammation can all support our bodies' natural healing processes. Always remember to drink lots of water, pay attention to what your body requires, and modify your diet gradually. We may become the captains of our own health and lead vibrant lives if we adopt a balanced and attentive approach. My buddies, it's time to get dressed up and show off!

Foods to Avoid

As a medical practitioner and health and wellness coach, I have witnessed some truly eye-opening things when it comes to diverticulitis management. The impact that nutrition and lifestyle choices may have is astounding. To be completely honest, there isn't a single treatment plan that works for everyone when it comes to this issue. However, I can assure you that some foods have the potential to exacerbate your symptoms and set off those excruciating flare-ups. Fortunately, you can find a great deal of relief if you can identify these triggers and make some focused dietary changes.

Let's now discuss the most important one: fibre. It's essential to diverticulitis management. You see, maintaining regular bowel movements and avoiding constipation—a significant risk factor for diverticulitis—requires consuming adequate fibre. The problem is that not every fibre is made equally. In fact, certain kinds of fibre may exacerbate your symptoms.

Soluble fibre can be found in foods such as fruits, beans, and oats. The reason this thing works so well is that it generates a gel-like substance that aids in proper digestion. It's generally well tolerated and may even provide relief from symptoms like gas and bloating. On the other hand, insoluble fibre can be found in vegetables, nuts, and whole grains. This fibre can raise the pressure inside your intestines and give your stool more volume. And if you have diverticulitis, that's unfortunate because it can trigger inflammation and excruciating flare-ups.

Consider entire grains as an example. Although they're frequently promoted as being incredibly healthful, they actually contain a lot of insoluble fibre and can cause serious problems for those who have diverticulitis. Making the switch to refined grains with the insoluble fibre removed, such as white rice or bread, may help some people. To be clear, however, refining grains also entails removing vital nutrients, and that's detrimental to your long-term health. As an alternative, I'd advise looking at soluble fiber-rich foods like brown rice, quinoa, or even gluten-free alternatives like buckwheat or amaranth.

Nuts and seeds are next on the attack list. Don't get me wrong, they are incredibly nutrient-dense, however people who have diverticulitis may find their high fibre and fat content quite bothersome. To make matters worse, those tiny devils with their sharp edges have the potential to become lodged in those diverticula. Therefore, it's advisable to avoid nuts and seeds, particularly when experiencing flare-ups. But fear not—you may still satisfy your nutty cravings with seedless substitutes like tahini or sunflower butter, or with nut butters.

Let's get spicy now! Hold on, forget that. You should avoid eating spicy meals if you have diverticulitis. Foods like curries, hot sauces, and chilli peppers can significantly agitate your body and exacerbate your symptoms. These foods contain a troublesome ingredient called capsaicin, which has the potential to aggravate your gut and increase inflammation. For that reason, if you enjoy a little kick in your food, consider substituting milder herbs or spices. It's still flavorful without adding to your agony.

I don't know about you, but I adore dishes that are heavy in fat. Sadly, these people should be avoided completely or kept to a minimum when it comes to diverticulitis. You ask, why? These fatty treats can be difficult to digest and severely damage your gut. Moreover, gaining weight due to excess fat raises the likelihood of experiencing additional episodes of diverticulitis. Therefore, use healthy cooking techniques like baking, grilling, or steaming, and stick to lean protein sources like skinless chicken or fish. Your stomach will appreciate it.

Let's finally discuss alcohol and caffeine. I won't advise you to throw them out entirely, but it's better to use them sparingly, if at all. Caffeine and alcohol have a strong inflammatory effect on the stomach and can disrupt digestion. Furthermore, they have the potential to dehydrate you, which is really harmful when it comes to diverticulitis. Thus, make an effort to stay hydrated by drinking lots of water. As a better option, consider trying a tasty herbal tea or infused water.

That's all there is to it, friend. Choosing foods mindfully can have a significant impact on how you manage your diverticulitis. Pay attention to the high-fiber foods that won't aggravate your condition further, stay away from those bothersome triggers, and substitute healthier options. How much better you may feel and how much more power you have over your life will astound you. Of course, the best people to ask for individualised counsel based on your needs and medical history are your healthcare physician or a licenced dietitian.

Meal Planning and Recipes

As a physician and health coach, I frequently field a barrage of inquiries from diverticulitis patients. They frequently ask me how to prepare meals that will both help their bodies heal and lessen their symptoms. Thus, I will walk you through meal planning step-by-step in this part and present some delicious dishes that are ideal for anyone with diverticulitis.

Organizing your meals is essential for treating diverticulitis. It enables us to ensure that the foods we eat provide us with all the essential nutrients we require to be healthy while also being easy on our digestive systems. We may repair those bothersome diverticula, reduce inflammation, and strengthen our entire body by adhering to a thoughtful meal plan.

Alright, let's begin with Step 1: learning about the meals that are healthy for you in the event that you have diverticulitis. Keep in mind that each person is unique, therefore you may have dietary limits or intolerances to certain foods. However, in general, I can provide you some guidelines that may be useful.

First, meals high in fibre. You need to consume enough fibre to help your bowels function properly and prevent constipation. Choose whole grains, legumes, fruits, and vegetables that are high in fibre but also gentle on the stomach.

Lean proteins come next. They are necessary for providing your body with all the essential amino acids it needs and for mending tissue. Tofu, fish, poultry, and lentils are your friends when it comes to lean protein.

Remember the importance of healthy fats as well. Not only are they beneficial to your health in general, but they can help reduce inflammation. Thus, your heroes can be foods like avocados, almonds, seeds, and olive oil.

And you want to eat foods high in probiotics to take care of your gut. These are the kinds of meals that are rich in beneficial bacteria that aid in digestion. Savor foods high in probiotics, such as yoghurt, kefir, sauerkraut, and kimchi.

Now that we know which foods are safe for people with diverticulitis, let's move on to Step 2: some useful advice for meal planning that will make your life even easier.

Firstly, make a plan in advance. Set aside some time at the beginning of each week to plan your meals. In this manner, you'll maintain organisation and guarantee that all the necessary elements are on hand.

Second, variation is what makes life interesting. Try to incorporate a variety of foods in your meals so that you can get as many different kinds of nutrients as possible. Everything will taste better that way, and you'll be consuming all the healthy nutrients your body needs.

Thirdly, let's talk about wonderful stuff: create large quantities. Make a large batch of anything delicious, such as soup or roasted vegetables, and freeze it for later. In this manner, you won't have to slave over the stove all day long to have something nutritious to eat.

Fourth on the list: leftovers, yum! None of such wonderful stuff should be wasted. Use your imagination and come up with numerous uses for your leftovers. Chicken that you grilled last night? Add it to a salad or use it as a filler for wraps. Donate not, need not!

And lastly, tip number five: add some flavour! Up the ante on your dishes by utilising herbs and spices. Not only do they taste fantastic, but your diverticulitis will appreciate their anti-inflammatory properties.

Okay, things are moving along! Proceed to Step 3 now: I've created several incredibly nourishing recipes that are ideal for people who have diverticulitis. They taste fantastic and are loaded with all the good stuff we've been talking about.

First up, a smoothie bowl full with fibre. For added fibre, blend together frozen berries, spinach, ripe banana, almond milk, and ground flaxseeds. For a little crunch, sprinkle some sliced almonds or chia seeds over top. Mmmm!

We're going to serve quinoa salad with roasted vegetables next. Cook the quinoa, allow it to cool, and then toss it with the olive oil and herb-dressed roasted zucchini, bell peppers, and cherry tomatoes. Use a straightforward lemon vinaigrette to finish it off. What a taste explosion!

I've prepared grilled salmon with quinoa and steamed vegetables for those of you seafood enthusiasts. Add some herbs to the salmon, toss it on the grill, and serve it with some cooked quinoa on the side and some steamed broccoli or asparagus. It's a gourmet feast for your stomach!

Not to be overlooked is a substantial soup made with lentils and vegetables. Add the onions, garlic, and bell peppers along with a mixture of carrots, celery, and other veggies and sauté until soft. After adding some cooked lentils and vegetable stock, boil everything for a while until the flavours combine, then add your preferred herbs and spices. I refer to that as soup for the soul.

To sum up, meal planning is a huge help in controlling diverticulitis and maintaining overall health in your body. Meal planning can help you prepare meals that will help you heal and reduce symptoms. Here are some simple guidelines to help you get started. Thus, don't put it off any longer. Plan your meals in advance and get ready for a happy, contented tummy. You can do this!

Supplements and Nutritional Support

I've always believed in the potential of holistic healthcare and wellness, and I practise medicine as well as coaching health and wellbeing. Let me tell you, in my experience, when people plan their diets, seek counselling, make lifestyle changes, and learn self-care practises, their lives take on amazing transformations. It's incredible how these techniques can raise someone's quality of life. Furthermore, I firmly believe that a holistic approach that incorporates nutritional assistance and vitamins can significantly improve the course of diverticulitis.

Thus, we're delving into the world of supplements and their potential to aid in the management of diverticulitis in this chapter. I'll provide you with knowledge backed by research to enable you to decide if taking supplements is the best move for you. But keep in mind that supplements cannot replace a healthy diet or sound medical advice. Consult your healthcare professional before beginning a new supplement regimen.

To begin with, fibre. One of the most important aspects of controlling diverticulitis is maintaining regular bowel movements and avoiding colon inflammation. Fiber is also our covert weapon. It gives our stool more volume and facilitates its easy passage through our intestines. Constipation can occur when we don't consume enough fibre, which exacerbates the symptoms of diverticulitis.

You can think considering taking supplements if you're concerned about getting adequate fibre. Psyllium husk is an excellent choice. It is a soluble fibre that in our intestines transforms into a gel-like material. This softens the stool and encourages frequent bowel motions, which facilitate easier passage. It also lessens the chance of diverticulitis-related complications.

Methylcellulose is an additional bulk-forming fibre supplement. It forms that same gel-like substance in our intestines when we take it in. This gives our stools more volume, which helps to relieve the symptoms of diverticulitis and avoid constipation.

The omega-3 fatty acids are the next topic. Diverticulitis is largely caused by inflammation, and omega-3s have incredible anti-inflammatory qualities. They are present in flaxseeds and chia seeds, as well as fatty seafood like salmon, mackerel, and sardines.

But taking a fish oil supplement could be the best option if you're having trouble getting enough omega-3s in your diet. They provide you with all the omega-3 fatty acids required to lessen colon inflammation, and they are generally accessible.

Let's now discuss the microorganisms in our stomachs. They are essential for gut health, and diverticulitis can result from an imbalance. That's the role of probiotics. When we eat enough of these living bacteria and yeasts, our bodies can benefit in a variety of ways. They lessen inflammation and support gut health by assisting in the restoration of the natural balance of our gut flora.

Bifidobacterium and Lactobacillus are two probiotic strains that have been researched in relation to diverticulitis. These tiny creatures help with constipation, gas, and bloating. They are present in meals like fermented vegetables and yoghurt. If those don't appeal to you, however, a probiotic supplement might.

Let's now discuss vitamin D in more detail. Our bodies create this vitamin, which is frequently referred to as the "sunshine vitamin," when we are exposed to sunlight. The major functions of vitamin D are to support and maintain bone health and the immune system. And here's the thing: a recent study connected a low level of vitamin D to a higher risk of diverticulitis. Therefore, your healthcare professional may recommend a vitamin D supplement if you don't get enough sun exposure or if your vitamin D levels are low. It will keep you at the same level, promoting general health and maybe lowering the chance of diverticular issues.

Not to be overlooked is turmeric. This bright yellow spice, which you have undoubtedly seen before, is well known for having anti-inflammatory qualities. Curcumin is the turmeric's hidden component. Curcumin has been the subject of years of research and has demonstrated some genuine promise in lowering colon inflammation and easing the symptoms of diverticulitis.

Adding turmeric to your food can be as easy as making turmeric tea or adding it to your favourite recipes. If you don't think you're receiving enough, you can take a supplement that contains curcumin.

In summary, nutritional support and supplements can be effective methods for controlling diverticulitis. However, keep in mind that they cannot replace a well-balanced diet or medical guidance. Consider them a component of an all-encompassing strategy that consists of frequent check-ups, a balanced diet, and lifestyle modifications.

As with any new supplement regimen, make sure to consult your physician first. They will assist you in determining whether it is appropriate for your particular needs and safe. They can advise you on the appropriate dosage and duration of supplementation.

In summary, incorporating fibre, probiotics, omega-3 fatty acids, vitamin D, and turmeric into your diverticulitis treatment regimen can improve your general health and lower your chance of problems. Recall that the key to making the most of your diverticulitis life is managing your health and collaborating with a group of medical professionals.

Hydration and Digestive Health

My friends, let's talk about being hydrated. You know, it's all about providing your body with adequate fluids to maintain optimal health. As you can see, water makes up an astounding 60% of our body weight, making it the MVP of our systems. It serves as, essentially, the gasoline that keeps everything operating properly. Therefore, when we discuss being hydrated, we are referring to ensuring that our bodies have an enough amount of water to support life.

And believe me when I say that maintaining adequate water is crucial for the health of our digestive systems. You see, water is necessary for the movement and absorption of all the vital nutrients that we put into our body. Let's just say that things can get a bit blocked up when we don't give it enough water. It is possible that you will have symptoms such as bloating, constipation, and overall discomfort. Not enjoyable at all, my friends, not enjoyable at all.

Therefore, staying hydrated is even more crucial when a person has diverticulitis, which is an infection or inflammation of pouches that occur in the colon. It feels like a complete gut check when those flare-ups occur. At such point, adequate hydration can truly be life-saving. It can assist in reducing the discomfort associated with those symptoms as well as preventing further bouts from negatively impacting your health.

In fact, research has shown that dehydration might exacerbate diverticulitis symptoms. Your faeces may become tougher and much more challenging to pass when your body is dehydrated. Not to mention, being dehydrated might interfere with your colon's blood flow, making it more difficult for it to recover from all that inflammation. Yeah, it's scary.

The good news is here, though, my friends. It feels good to give your gut a high five when you're drinking enough water. It can support both the smooth operation of your stool and the flow of stuff. And life is much more comfortable when you're not stressing your diverticula.

Furthermore, a well-hydrated colon helps prevent difficulties and heal more quickly. It gives your digestive system superpowers.

In order to stay in the game of hydration, how much water should you be drinking? Nowadays, the sophisticated people advise aiming for eight 8-ounce glasses each day at the very least. That is equivalent to two litres or half a gallon. Let's not get too hung up on the figures, though. Since every person is different, factors such as age, degree of exercise, and even the weather can affect how much water you require. So, my friends, pay attention to your bodies and sip away when you feel thirsty.

Here's a little insider advice for you right now. Consuming foods high in water content can be your best ally in the fight against dehydration. Consider refreshing fruits such as cucumbers, oranges, and watermelon. Water power is all over them. Remember to include broths and soups as well. They may also provide you with an additional hydration boost.

Hey, I understand, but. It can be difficult to stay hydrated, particularly when those annoying flare-ups happen. It's as if your thirst and hunger simply vanish. Friends, that's where a health and wellness coach really shines. They can design a customised hydration regimen particularly for you, acting as your own hydration superhero.

Being aware of how much water you consume is one tip they could offer. That entails monitoring your daily alcohol use, including when and how much you drink. Maybe set a reminder or two and keep that water bottle handy. Friends, it all comes down to consciously trying to keep hydrated.

Yes, and it all comes down to time. Try drinking water throughout the day rather than all at once. Your body will be able to absorb and utilise it more effectively in this manner. Your stomach will appreciate it, I promise.

Let's now discuss a few delicious drinks. Herbal teas, such as ginger or peppermint, can treat your digestive tract to a spa day. All of them are calming and can lessen cramping and bloating. Just use caution when consuming sodas and other caffeinated beverages. They may act as nuisances, causing discomfort and aggravating your condition.

In summary, when you have diverticulitis, staying hydrated is like having the magic ingredient for a happy stomach. It all comes down to providing your body with the water it requires to process those nutrients, stay hydrated, and repair itself during episodes of inflammation. So get ready to feel fantastic from the inside out by working with a health and wellness coach to create a personalised hydration strategy that suits your needs. My friends, let's toast to a belly that is well hydrated!

Mindful Eating and Emotional Well-Being

Friends, let's chat about mindful eating. Imagine yourself sitting down at the table and giving the act of eating your whole attention. No interruptions, no condemnation. Just you and your meal, coexisting harmoniously. As you can see, a lot of us have forgotten how to cook. Food is shovelled into our mouths without being fully chewed or appreciated for its flavours. It's also having a negative impact on our hearts in addition to our waistlines.

We eat on the move since we live in such a hectic and fast-paced world. As we browse through social media or respond to emails, we stuff our faces. However, distancing ourselves from the act of eating can cause mental havoc and result in emotional eating and a negative relationship with food. Let's introduce mindful eating. It all comes down to making mindful eating decisions and living in the present.

Emotional well-being can be greatly enhanced by mindful eating. Research indicates that when we focus on our food, we experience more satisfaction. Every flavour is dancing on your taste buds, creating the impression of a party in your tongue. Furthermore, when we take our time and enjoy our food, our bodies truly let us know when we are satisfied. My friends, let's stop this pointless cramming. Balance and weight control are key in this dance, particularly for people who have diverticulitis.

However, it goes beyond our bodily well-being. Emotional health also benefits from mindful eating. It's about accepting a healthy relationship with our body and being grateful for the sustenance that food gives us. No strict regulations or guilt trips anymore. By practising mindfulness in our eating habits, we may let go of external constraints and pay attention to our bodies' needs. It feels like a warm, consoling hug from the inside out for ourselves.

It's time to discuss some tactics, my friends who enjoy eating. Pay attention to your body first. Before you dig in, ask yourself if you're actually hungry or if you're just bored or worried. Throughout your meal, be mindful of your feelings. Take note of any modifications to your bodily experiences. And set down your fork, my friend, as soon as you're satisfied. After that, pause to consider. Did your dinner satisfy you? Did it fuel your body and give you a happy smile?

Oh, and let's not overlook those scents, tastes, and sensations. Make use of all of your senses. Chew on every bite as though it's the greatest thing you've ever had. Observe how the flavour and texture develop in your mouth. Hey, enjoy the flavours and colours of your cuisine. Let it be a celebration of life and a feast for the senses.

Not to mention, when it comes to eating, we need to make a safe zone for ourselves. Put an end to designating food as "good" or "evil." Now is the time to let go of the shame and guilt. Food is designed to fuel us, my friends, and a well-balanced diet can include a wide variety of delectable foods.

And keep in mind that emotional well-being encompasses more than just mindful eating. Breathe deeply, engage in meditation, or simply write everything on your mind in a journal. Seek out a network of support, be it a support group, a therapist, or fellow travellers. To fully control your diverticulitis and attain mental well-being, my friends, it takes a community.

As a physician and wellness coach, you see, I've seen it all. I have seen firsthand the transformational power of mindful eating on our bodies and minds. You may nourish your body and soul and develop a better relationship with food by implementing these ideas into your daily life. Thus, keep in mind, my friends, that inner mending begins. Eating with awareness is the key to living a life worth living.

Medical Interventions and Treatment Approaches

Medication Management

Alright, let's discuss this illness known as diverticulitis. Imagine that the diverticula, which are pouches found in your colon, become irritated or infected when that happens. And boy, can the symptoms be variable; in addition to a slight discomfort, you may experience severe abdominal pain, fever, and even complications such as perforations or abscesses. That sounds like fun.

Currently, diverticulitis management is not easy. It's imperative to address the pain, infection, and inflammation directly while also preventing further flare-ups. Medication management then becomes relevant.

We need to take care of that inflammation first. Nonsteroidal anti-inflammatory medicines (NSAIDs), such as naproxen or ibuprofen, come to the rescue. These little creatures can assist in lessening intestinal discomfort and inflammation. But be careful when using these guys—long-term use may cause unintended problems including kidney damage or gastrointestinal bleeding. Therefore, make sure a healthcare expert is helping you and refrain from going beyond.

Now, antibiotics may become your new best friend when things get really hot or when complications like perforations or abscesses appear. These medications are suggested to eradicate those bothersome bacterial infections and prevent them from causing more damage. It's likely that you'll hear terms like ciprofloxacin and metronidazole mentioned a lot because they work well to eradicate those germs and encourage recovery. Just make sure you complete the entire course of medicines as directed by your physician in order to permanently eradicate that infection.

Oh, and don't forget about taking care of those adorable diverticulitis symptoms. One of the most common ones is stomach pain, which may require the use of opioids or acetaminophen as an analgesic. But don't worry, opioids are serious drugs; use them under a doctor's supervision to prevent addiction or reliance.

And how could we overlook the delight of loose stools or diarrhoea? Who doesn't enjoy that, really? You can use antidiarrheal drugs, such as loperamide, to slow down that crazy ride. They'll ease the situation and provide you with much-needed comfort. But keep in mind, you shouldn't just take those medications and go to bed. Instead of depending only on antidiarrheal medications in the long run, you will need to address the underlying cause of the diarrhoea.

There is much to consider when it comes to using medicine to treat diverticulitis. First of all, get a close friend who works in healthcare. They will evaluate the particulars of your case and choose the most appropriate course of treatment. Your medical history, the severity of your diverticulitis, and any additional medications you are taking will all be considered. You're under capable care!

Not to mention the bothersome side effects that medications may have. Certain prescriptions can come with unexpected side effects. For example, NSAIDs can cause problems with your kidneys or gastrointestinal tract, while opioids can lead to a host of exciting addiction and dependency issues. The issue is, though, if you and your healthcare provider have an honest and open channel of communication, they will make sure that the advantages of the medication outweigh the hazards. You are protected by them.

Hey, let's not limit ourselves to medication. Making certain lifestyle changes, organising your food, seeking counselling, and engaging in self-care practises are essential to defeating diverticulitis. Merely taking medication won't solve the underlying cause of the issue or put an end to flare-ups. Thus, take care of your diet, exercise, stress management, and don't be embarrassed to ask for help when you need it. This all-encompassing strategy will improve the effectiveness of those medications and elevate your overall result.

To put it briefly, treating diverticulitis entails calling in the medicine cavalry. They'll quickly arrive, take care of the infection and inflammation, and lessen the discomfort caused by those symptoms.

However, keep in mind to use those medications under the supervision of a healthcare professional, be aware of any potential adverse effects, and combine them with lifestyle modifications and self-care practises. You will be living your best life and kicking diverticulitis to the curb together.

Surgical Options and Considerations

Now, let us discuss diverticulitis. It's this bothersome disorder where the small pouches along the wall of your colon called diverticula become inflamed or infected. Let me tell you, it's not exactly a party in there. In certain situations, you can control it with dietary adjustments, relaxation, and medication. On occasion, however, surgery is the best option.

Now, let me explain before you start seeing a scenario from Grey's Anatomy. Diverticulitis surgery is a serious medical procedure. There are numerous reasons why it is advised. For example, if you experience recurrent episodes or severe consequences such as fistulas or abscesses. You may end up on the surgical table even if you have a ruptured colon.

There are several options available when it comes to surgery. It all depends on how dire things are and how well you're feeling overall. A bowel resection is one frequent operation. Your colon's damaged section is removed, and the remaining portion is reconnected. A large incision can be made, or sophisticated laparoscopic or robotically assisted methods can be used.

Hold on, though—more. there's A colostomy is an additional choice. Yes, they make a cut in your abdomen and attach a bag to it. It may not be the most attractive picture, but it effectively removes all waste from your colon. This is for situations in which a bowel resection is not appropriate or in which you require a brief hiatus to allow the condition to heal. Colostomies can be either permanent or temporary, depending on the circumstances.

Now, you need to have a serious conversation with your healthcare staff before you blindly walk into the operating room. It's a decision with many moving parts. How many times a day is ruined by this condition? To what extent does it affect your standard of living? What are the advantages and disadvantages of surgery? Heck, how's your general health these days? You need to go deep with your team to determine what's best for you. The ultimate goal is to lessen any dangerous business and improve your long-term well-being.

There's a catch, though. Like any other procedure, surgery has hazards. Infections, haemorrhage, clots, and even harm to other organs are possible. Thus, understanding what you're entering into is essential. The worst part is that having a knowledgeable surgeon can really make a difference. They can ensure that everything goes as well as possible for you and reduce the likelihood of problems.

Here's the thing: your general health must be taken into account while deciding whether to get surgery. Your age, any underlying medical conditions, and other risk factors may all have an impact on how well the treatment goes. Before they perform their magic in the operating room, you may occasionally need to get your health in the best possible shape.

In summary, surgery is a viable option for treating diverticulitis. Surgery could be your best option for relief if the conservative measures don't work or if things become too complicated. Just make sure you have a genuine heart-to-heart with your healthcare staff, discussing all the advantages and disadvantages. For those with diverticulitis, surgery can be a game-changer if done correctly, with the right skills, and with consideration for your needs.

Alternative Therapies and Complementary Approaches

Okay, so the standard medical approach to treating diverticulitis usually entails taking antibiotics, adhering to a bland liquid diet, and taking some painkillers. Indeed, those measures are crucial for managing the infection and relieving your digestive tract, but there are additional remedies you can attempt in addition to them. You know, complementary and alternative therapies can really give you that extra push to feel better and maintain overall well-being.

Acupuncture is one alternative therapy that has recently attracted a lot of interest. It's probably not unfamiliar to you; it's a practise from ancient Chinese medicine in which extremely thin needles are inserted into specific body locations. It may sound extreme, but evidence indicates that when you have diverticulitis, it can assist to relieve discomfort, improve your bowel movements, and lower inflammation. It appears that it realigns your body's equilibrium and Qi (pronounced "chee"), or energy flow, which is precisely what your body needs to heal.

And now for something else you should look into: herbal medicine. Mother Nature has provided us with an abundance of plants and herbs that offer remarkable health advantages. I am referring, among other things, to marshmallow root, licorice root, and slippery elm. These herbs have long been used to treat a variety of digestive problems and to soothe the old digestive system. They can aid in the healing of your intestinal lining, have anti-inflammatory qualities, and—best of all—offer some respite from the persistent soreness and pain in your belly. Just keep in mind that it's a good idea to find a qualified herbalist or naturopathic doctor who can ensure everything is in order before venturing too far into the realm of herbs. You should use caution while combining certain plants with prescription drugs.

And remember, there's a connection between your mind and body. Your diverticulitis may truly go completely crazy if you have ongoing stress and worry. Thus, it could be worthwhile to try yoga and meditation. It's true that these techniques can help you de-stress, unwind, and enhance your general wellbeing. It all comes down to developing inner resilience and serenity, which can improve both your mental and digestive health.

Let's talk about food now. As everyone knows, you have to take it easy and stick to the clear liquid diet during those flare-ups. However, you can completely alter your eating habits in the long run to stop these relapses. The best diet is one that consists mostly of whole, high-fiber foods. Consider lean proteins, whole grains, legumes, and fruits and vegetables. They supply all the essential nutrients your body requires to be in optimal condition and maintain regular bowel motions. Furthermore, remember to include probiotics in your daily regimen. You already know how crucial a balanced gut flora is to healthy digestion and general well-being. These little fellas maintain that equilibrium.

Finding strategies to manage stress is essential because it can be a major pain in the you-know-what. Have a conversation with a psychologist or counsellor. They can assist you in addressing any emotional problems that may be interfering with your physical well-being. In addition, they will assist you in cultivating a cheerful outlook and some lovely coping mechanisms. Who doesn't need that in their life, let's face it?

Alright, let me tell you about a few more awesome self-care activities. Would you mind massaging your abdomen? It facilitates bowel movement, improves blood flow, and really reduces pain and suffering. Remember the benefits of hot and cold therapy as well. To relieve yourself of the discomfort and minimise inflammation, heat up a heating pad or apply some ice packs. You can apply herbal compresses, such as chamomile or ginger ones, to your stomach to help soothe it. If you're up for an extreme adventure, you could even try hydrotherapy. You know, soaking in various forms and temps of water to help you relax and ease your pain.

Finally, but most importantly, you need to learn coping mechanisms for living with diverticulitis and its effects on your daily routine. I realise it's not easy. Both physically and psychologically, having a chronic illness has its costs. Therefore, cultivate a support network of understanding individuals, make sure you have hobbies that help you stay sane, practise self-care like a boss, and never be afraid to ask for professional help when you need it. I promise you, you need to pay attention to your body, be aware of your boundaries, and seek for help when you need it. Managing diverticulitis and regaining control over your general health can be achieved by combining these complementary and alternative methods with your usual medical care.

All things considered, it's very evident that complementary and alternative therapies can be extremely beneficial in treating diverticulitis. We have herbal medication, acupuncture, mindfulness practises like yoga and meditation, food modifications, stress management measures, self-care skills, and coping mechanisms that work for you. It's important to focus on healing, feeling better, and reaching a point where you can live in addition to simply treating the symptoms. Life of Yours. Thus, don't be scared to do these things, but make sure you're working with a healthcare professional who is knowledgeable and capable of guiding you through the process in a safe and efficient manner. Embrace the full picture, my friend, and you'll discover that life can truly be wonderful—even if diverticulitis is your buddy.

Preventive Measures and Lifestyle Modifications

You know, I really think that prevention is crucial when it comes to managing diverticulitis and avoiding any unpleasant complications. You can take control of your health and be proactive, so why wait for something to go wrong? My goal as a physician and health coach is to arm you with all the information and resources you need to effectively treat diverticulitis.

Thus, in this brief part, I will guide you through a methodical process of implementing lifestyle modifications that will not only prevent difficulties but also improve your overall well-being. We will cover everything, including how you exercise, what you eat, and how you cope with stress. My friend, it's a total package deal.

Let's start by discussing how important it is to have routine checkups. These check-ups with your doctor can identify any possible problems early on and save you a great deal of hassle. They can also offer you advice on how to modify your lifestyle in light of your particular ailment. Accept the occasional trip to the doctor; it will be worthwhile.

The exciting part is here: the food. For diverticulitis, a high-fiber diet is going to be your best friend. It keeps your digestive tract working freely, avoids constipation, and eases the strain on those bothersome diverticula. So fill your plate high with whole grains, legumes, fruits, and vegetables. Your stomach will appreciate it.

Oh, and remember to drink plenty of water. It's like offering your digestive system a helping hand when you drink adequate water. It prevents constipation, softens your faeces, and keeps things moving. Try to consume eight glasses of water or more each day. Let's toast to it!

Let's now discuss how to start your body moving. Frequent exercise not only improves general health but also significantly improves diverticulitis management. You just need to start exercising for at least 30 minutes most days of the week; you don't need to become an avid gym goer or anything. Go for a swim, go for a brisk walk, jump on your bike, or do whatever else you enjoy to get your heart rate up.

Alright, let's discuss stress. It can make things worse, as we all know. Diverticulitis is not an exception, though. Therefore, learning effective stress management techniques will be essential in the long run. Try practising yoga, deep breathing techniques, meditation, or simply just doing what you enjoy. Anything that eases your tension and promotes relaxation will work.

Another small secret for you to know is that probiotics will be your allies in the battle against diverticulitis. These microorganisms are beneficial bacteria that support intestinal health. Foods such as yoghurt, kefir, sauerkraut, and kimchi contain them. Your doctor can supply you with vitamins if you require further support.

Alright, have a seat; this one may not go as planned. Certain meals have the ability to trigger an exacerbation of your diverticulitis. You know the drill: processed foods, spicy foods, refined cereals, and anything heavy in saturated fats. Yes, I realise this is a bit of a buzzkill, but believe me when I say that staying away from these bad guys will prevent severe flare-ups and inflammation. Thus, perhaps keep a meal journal and record what triggers those symptoms.

On to the beverages now. Overindulgence in caffeine and alcohol can severely damage your digestive tract and exacerbate your diverticulitis. So, perhaps we should cut back on our alcohol consumption and forgo that third cup of coffee. I swear, your stomach will appreciate it.

Hey, let's take a moment to discuss weight control. Maintaining a healthy weight is crucial for the treatment of diverticulitis. Having excess weight might strain your digestive system and increase the likelihood of problems. But don't be alarmed, buddy. You can conquer this with regular exercise and a healthy diet. You can do this.

But hey, let's not forget about the emotional side of things. Suffering from a chronic illness such as diverticulitis can be emotionally taxing. Seeking much-needed support from friends, family, or a support group shouldn't be a source of fear. It is also OK to speak with a mental health professional if you require professional assistance. They have all the advice you need to deal with the emotional aspect of things.

Through these actions and adjustments, you will significantly lower the likelihood of problems and enhance your general quality of life. Recall that proactive and persistent management is key. Speak with your healthcare practitioner, who can assist you in customising these tactics to meet your needs and creating a strategy that suits you.

We will delve even further into diverticulitis therapies in the upcoming chapter. We'll look at complementary therapy in addition to the traditional stuff. We'll figure out the finest strategies to help you handle this and have the best possible life, I promise. So, my friend, stay put. We can handle this.

Recovery and Rehabilitation

You recently underwent surgery or some other medical intervention, then? Let me tell you, though: the road to rehabilitation is far from easy. It's a fact that your body requires time to mend itself. Numerous factors, including the type of treatment you received and your general state of health, will affect how long it takes you to recover. One thing is certain, though: you must prioritise self-care and pay attention to your medical team.

Now, controlling your pain is crucial to your recuperation. You want to be as comfortable as possible as your body works its magic, I promise. Your medical team will provide you with an individualised pain management strategy that may involve medication, physical therapy, and other advanced treatments.

Physical therapy, by the way, will play a major role in your healing process. The physical therapy team will perform miracles and assist you in getting back on your feet. To increase your strength, flexibility, and other desirable qualities, they will have you perform workouts and procedures. They'll get you moving again, whether they're working on your entire body or just a particular area that was impacted by the treatment.

However, my friend, don't go thinking you can spend the entire day lounging on the couch. It all comes down to striking a balance between activity and rest. Although you must get enough sleep, spending too much time on the couch can worsen your situation. Your medical staff will advise you on the appropriate amount of exercise, escalating the level of intensity as your strength improves.

Now, mental health is just as important to recovery as physical health. Throughout the entire healing process, emotions can run amok—trust me, I've been there. Feeling vulnerable, depressed, and anxious are all included in the package. Counseling and psychological strategies can help with it. You can recover emotionally and receive major therapeutic benefits from talking things out in a secure environment.

Furthermore, complimentary approaches can transform the game if you're willing to try them. Relaxation techniques, meditation, mindfulness—anything that keeps your mind clear and helps you handle stress—are all beneficial. My friend, it all comes down to figuring out what works for you.

Now, though, what? You are the captain of your own rehabilitation, not just a passenger. It's a big power move to take charge of your own recovery. You can modify your way of life by doing things like eating a better diet or working out frequently. And remember to take care of yourself. No matter what, you should prioritise your well-being and relaxation.

It's not easy, my buddy, to deal with the psychological and emotional aftermath of recovery. However, I can assure you that there are coping mechanisms available to assist you in getting through difficult times. Rely on your family and friends, join online forums or support groups, and don't forget to use your creative outlets. You will grow stronger as you ride these waves more often.

Not to be overlooked is the importance of communication with your healthcare staff. Inform them of any concerns and schedule routine check-ups to keep them informed. They'll support you at every turn and modify your treatment plan as necessary.

Remind yourself that you are the only one going through this treatment and recovery process. Treat yourself with kindness, patience, and respect for your body. You're putting yourself in a position to have a long and healthy future by making self-care a priority, getting involved in your rehabilitation, and asking for help when you need it.

We'll discuss dietary advice and lifestyle modifications for my fellow diverticulitis fighters in the upcoming chapter. You can take charge of your health and put an end to diverticulitis with these weapons in your toolbox. My friend, let's conquer this road together.

Patient-Centered Care and Advocacy

To begin with, allow me to share with you one of the main reasons I work as a medical doctor and health and wellness consultant. This idea is known as patient-centered care. And believe me when I say that it's revolutionary.

Imagine a healthcare strategy that considers the individual as a whole, including their values, beliefs, and preferences. It's important to genuinely understand the patient and involve them in the decision-making process rather than just treating symptoms with a band-aid solution. With the ultimate goal of achieving the best results for each individual, it's similar to a partnership between the patient and their healthcare practitioner.

Thus, patient-centered therapy becomes even more crucial for controlling diverticulitis. There is no one-size-fits-all treatment for diverticulitis. Everybody is unique, with their own set of circumstances, interests, and aspirations. Therefore, it's critical to modify the management techniques to meet the unique requirements of each patient.

And as you can see, I'm all about giving patients the tools they need to actively participate in their own medical care. In my opinion as a health and wellness coach, information is power. Therefore, it is my responsibility to ensure that patients are well informed about their disease, possible therapies, and expected outcomes. Equipped with this knowledge, patients may truly take control of their health and make educated decisions for themselves. Furthermore, patients who take an active role in their own care are far more likely to follow their treatment plans, alter their lifestyles, and have improved outcomes.

This is when things really start to get exciting: advocacy. Imagine yourself speaking up for someone when they are unable to do it for themselves. When it comes to managing diverticulitis, we require advocates at every stage. We must push for individualised and comprehensive care that addresses lifestyle modifications, mental health support, and self-care practises in addition to medical issues. Ensuring patients have access to a comprehensive team of professionals who can support them during this journey is crucial.

However, receiving the best care is only one aspect of it; another is ensuring that patients have access to the most recent research and evidence-based recommendations. It is my duty as a medical professional and health and wellness coach to be current on the most recent research regarding diverticulitis treatment in order to give my patients the best care possible. I also encourage my patients to seek out information, pose questions, and engage in candid discussions with their healthcare professionals.

And pay attention, I am aware that obstacles may occur on the path. Certain patients encounter obstacles such as restricted healthcare access, budgetary limitations, or insufficient social support. The fact is, though, that our purpose is to assist them in overcoming those challenges. We wish to see to it that they receive the attention they require and merit.

Thus, my friend, it all boils down to advocacy and empowerment. We empower people to take charge of their healthcare journeys by providing them with information and assistance. They take on the role of their own advocates, seeking the care that best suits their needs and making educated judgments. And what's this? Better results, happier patients, and a true sense of control over their health follow from this.

I will now go even further into methods and approaches in the upcoming chapters to assist you in adopting patient-centered care and advocacy in the treatment of diverticulitis. I'm here to help you every step of the way; trust me, there's a lot to unpack.

But before we go any further, let me discuss a few points that I believe are essential to the management of diverticulitis. Establishing a robust and affirmative rapport between the patient and their physician is a game-changer. It should be easy for patients to ask questions, voice concerns, and take an active role in their own care. The main goal is to establish a secure environment in which kids feel free to express themselves.

Integrating several disciplines and methodologies is another crucial component of diverticulitis care. This illness has an impact on a person's entire life, not simply their physical health. So, we can give patients a comprehensive support system by incorporating things like psychology, counselling, and self-care practises.

Naturally, we also need to consider making lifestyle and self-care changes. This entails planning a nutritious diet, exercising, reducing stress, and implementing practises like mindfulness and relaxation. Patients can effectively control their symptoms and reduce the likelihood of relapses when they are equipped with the self-care resources.

Not to mention, I want you to manage your own medical treatment. Seek second perspectives, make all of your questions answered, and take an active role in the process of making decisions. You can ensure that your requirements are satisfied and that your voice is heard by fighting for individualised and all-encompassing care.

That's the situation, my friend. Advocacy and patient-centered treatment are essential to the effective therapy of diverticulitis. Adopting these strategies helps us take an active role in our healthcare journey and fight for the treatment we are entitled to. So let's get together, give ourselves more power, and truly improve our lives.

Emerging Research and Innovations

Now, let us discuss diverticulitis. For years, medical professionals and researchers have been studying it in an effort to develop more effective treatments. And you know what? They've achieved some really remarkable advancements. With our increased knowledge of this illness, we may now better manage symptoms and guard against consequences.

The part that gut microbiota plays in diverticulitis is one area that has scientists really excited. I realise it seems very technical, but please be patient. The term "gut microbiota" refers to all of the bacteria and other microscopic creatures that inhabit our digestive tracts. And here's the thing: some astute individuals believe that diverticulitis may arise and worsen if there is an imbalance in these tiny creatures. Incredible, isn't it?

In fact, a research published in the Journal of Gastroenterology discovered that individuals with diverticulitis had higher concentrations of the harmful bacterium Escherichia coli in their digestive tracts than those without the illness. That's significant because it raises the possibility that we could develop new therapies that specifically target these gut bacteria. They're even researching probiotics, which you've certainly heard of, and prebiotics, which are essentially foods for the beneficial bacteria in your stomach. And, get ready for this... they're even researching a procedure known as faecal microbiota transplantation. Yes, you did hear me correctly. transplants of poop. Crazy, eh?

Let's now discuss an alternative method of treating diverticulitis: employing herbal medicines and natural supplements. You know, medical professionals frequently recommend surgery or prescription drugs, but each has drawbacks and hazards of its own. It follows that a large number of people are using alternative therapies to alleviate their symptoms and enhance their general health.

For instance, curcumin, a substance present in turmeric, was the subject of a research published in the Journal of Alternative and Complementary Medicine. And you know what? Due to its potent anti-inflammatory properties, curcumin has been shown to improve the symptoms of mild to moderate diverticulitis. Really neat, huh?

Not only that, though. An additional investigation into the impact of a combination of herbal extracts, such as peppermint and chamomile, on symptoms of diverticulitis was published in the Journal of Functional Foods. And you know what? In fact, this herbal mixture improved people's quality of life by reducing pain and inflammation. That is a significant victory, indeed.

Let me impart some knowledge to you now: these are all really exciting discoveries that give people with diverticulitis a glimpse of hope. Let's be realistic, though. To truly validate these findings and determine the most effective methods of utilising these herbs and supplements, more research is required.

Now, though, what? It's not just about supplements and herbal remedies. Nope, surgical treatment for diverticulitis has also shown significant breakthroughs. Laparoscopic surgery, also referred to as keyhole surgery, is a minimally invasive surgical technique. You know, to remove the problematic sections of the colon, doctors make smaller incisions and utilise tiny instruments and cameras instead of the enormous, terrifying ones. It resembles magic.

Why is this thing so awesome? Indeed, laparoscopic surgery is far superior to open surgery in the conventional sense. It translates into less discomfort, shortened hospital stays, and expedited recuperation. Furthermore, research has demonstrated that not only are there fewer issues, but the long-term results are also significantly superior. A win-win scenario exists.

And you know what else? The diagnostic and assessment of diverticulitis has completely changed as a result of our advanced imaging technology. Imaging techniques such as computed tomography (CT) scans and magnetic resonance imaging (MRI) are comparable to our arsenal's hidden weapons. These infants are able to identify diverticula, which are small sacs within the colon, as well as provide information about the level of inflammation and potential complications. It resembles superhuman vision.

But there's still more. Indeed, scientists have begun delving into the field of precision medicine, which is revolutionary. As you can see, the main goal of precision medicine is to customise care to each patient's particular genetic composition, way of life, and surroundings. It's similar to providing your body with the customised attention it truly needs.

This study examined genetic variants and their effect in diverticulitis, and it was published in the Journal of Personalized Medicine. And you know what? Certain markers that may indicate who is more likely to develop the illness were discovered. This implies that we can utilise this information to tailor treatment programmes to the specific needs of each patient. It is comparable to customised medicine.

Not to be overlooked is the potential of digital health technologies. This material is actually altering the game. Patients now have so much power thanks to telemedicine platforms, wearable technology, and applications. They have access to remote healthcare, progress tracking, and condition education. It's similar to bringing the doctor into your living room.

There you have it, then. We have hope and our approach to treating diverticulitis has changed because of all these incredible developments in the field. And that's fascinating material. By providing you with a comprehensive overview of the situation, I hope to empower you to make wise decisions for your own well-being. It is our responsibility as medical practitioners to remain abreast of these developments and to continue providing the best care that we can. It all comes down to treating the patient as a whole, mind and body.

www.ingramcontent.com/pod-product-compliance
Ingram Content Group Australia Pty Ltd
76 Discovery Rd, Dandenong South VIC 3175, AU
AUIIW011340280526
427809AU00034B/258

9 798223 760917